Redha Lakehal

Vascular trauma: clinical cases

Redha Lakehal

Vascular trauma: clinical cases

Vascular trauma

ScienciaScripts

Imprint
Any brand names and product names mentioned in this book are subject to trademark, brand or patent protection and are trademarks or registered trademarks of their respective holders. The use of brand names, product names, common names, trade names, product descriptions etc. even without a particular marking in this work is in no way to be construed to mean that such names may be regarded as unrestricted in respect of trademark and brand protection legislation and could thus be used by anyone.

Cover image: www.ingimage.com

This book is a translation from the original published under ISBN 978-620-3-44157-4.

Publisher:
Sciencia Scripts
is a trademark of
Dodo Books Indian Ocean Ltd. and OmniScriptum S.R.L Publishing group
Str. Armeneasca 28/1, office 1, Chisinau MD-2012, Republic of Moldova, Europe
Printed at: see last page
ISBN: 978-620-5-35549-7

Clinical case 01

Total transection of the humeral artery after a fall on a sharp part of a mirror: a case report.

Introduction :

Paediatric vascular injuries are rare, accounting for only about 0.6% to 2% of all traumatic paediatric injuries [1]. The most common mechanisms include road traffic accidents, firearm injuries, stab wounds and falls. The most frequently injured vessels are those of the upper limb, followed in decreasing frequency by abdominal vessels (inferior vena cava, iliac and renal vessels), vessels of the lower limbs, chest and neck [2,3].

Compared to adult vascular injuries, paediatric vascular injuries are more likely to be asymptomatic and are associated with vasospasm. Therefore, consideration of minor signs is essential. Minor signs require further diagnostic investigations such as Doppler ultrasound and/or CT angiography. Major signs warrant prompt intervention; these include persistent shock despite adequate resuscitation, active bleeding, rapidly expanding haematoma, decreased peripheral pulses, proximity of the wound path to major vessels and/or signs of nerve damage, arteriovenous fistula or distal ischaemia (pallor, pulselessness, paraesthesia and pain) [4,5].

The aim of this work is to show a domestic accident in a child, such as total section of the humeral artery by the sharp part of a mirror.

Observation:

We report the observation of an 08 year old girl who fell on a sharp part of a mirror without any bone lesion of the forearm with abolition of the left radial pulse without sensitivomotor disorders for more than 24 hours.

The physical examination revealed abolition of the radial pulse with coldness and pallor of the hand and forearm without sensory-motor deficit of the latter two.

The chest X-ray showed a TIA of 0.50.

The ECG was in regular sinus rhythm.

The patient was operated on under general anaesthesia with tracheal intubation in the supine position.

Intraoperative exploration found a 03 cm humeral arterial loss of substance with retracted and thrombosed ends without median nerve damage and without associated venous injury.

The procedure consisted of restoring humeral arterial continuity via the saphenous vein after preparation of the humeral arterial extremities with immobilisation of the upper limb by a plaster cast (Figures 1,2).

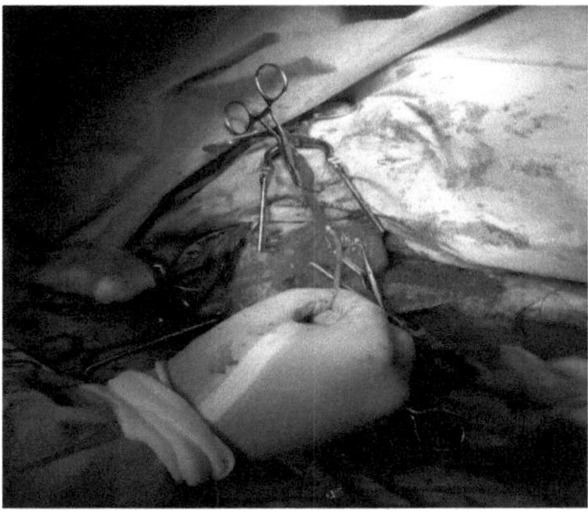

Figure 01: Intraoperative image during surgical exploration.

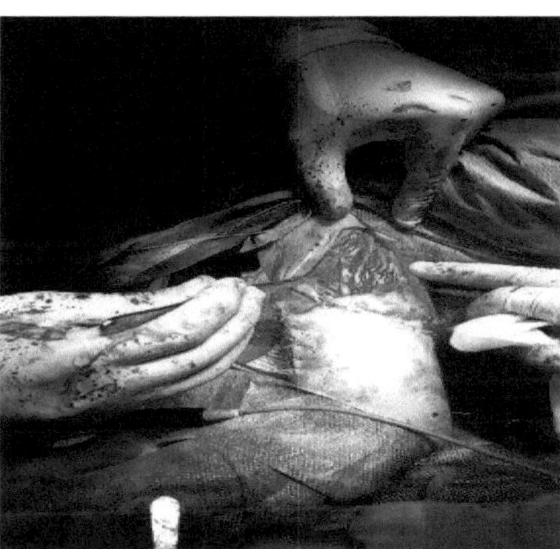

Figure 02: Intraoperative image after arterial reconstruction.

Results :

Postoperative follow-up was favourable in terms of revascularisation of the upper limb.

Stay in intensive care unit was 01 day.

The immediate and medium-term postoperative follow-up was favourable in terms of vitality and vascularity.

A follow-up CT angiogram of the traumatized limb at 06 months postoperatively showed a patent bypass without anastomotic stenosis.

Discussions :

Non-iatrogenic traumatic vascular injuries in children are rare and poorly published in the literature. Paediatric vascular injuries pose long-term problems mainly due to the continuous growth and development of children [1, 2, 3].

Although less frequent than in adults, a significant proportion were due to penetrating injuries. Vessels of the upper limb were the most frequently injured and were associated with low mortality. Injuries to the thoracic aorta were rare [4].

Blunt vascular injuries of the lower limbs most commonly occur in the anteroposterior tibial arteries; injured arteries of the proximal upper and lower limbs require resection with graft interposition, while those of the forearm or calf are usually ligated [5].

Appropriate treatment of children with acute arterial limb injuries requires early surgery and continuous postoperative follow-up during the growing years. The humeral arterial loss of substance was filled with a vascular substitute: saphenous vein in our patient. If chronic arterial insufficiency is observed, arteriograms should be performed and arterial reconstruction should be undertaken [6].

Despite the multidisciplinary diagnostic and treatment modalities available in paediatric trauma centres, traumatic vascular injury in children and adolescents is associated with significant morbidity and mortality in contemporary surgical practice [7] but lower than in adults [4].

However, the contemporary perioperative and long-term results after surgical revascularisation are excellent, as demonstrated in the series published by Wang SK and colleagues [8].

Conclusion:

Open vascular trauma can result in either haemorrhage or ischaemia. Exploration of the humeral artery must be systematic after open dislocation of the elbow. The presence of a vessel lesion must be suspected and explored in the presence of an opening in the path of a vascular axis.

Treatment is adapted to the vascular lesions and possibly to associated lesions. It is conventional surgical or endovascular. The urgency of its implementation depends on the intensity of the haemorrhagic shock or the downstream ischemic repercussions. Global complications arise from associated tendon and nerve injuries. Walkman's syndrome may occur postoperatively.

References:

1. Heinzerling NP, Sato TT. Pediatric Vascular Injuries. In: Dua A, Desai SS, Holcomb JB, Burgess AR, Freischlag JA, eds. Clinical Review of Vascular Trauma. Springer-Verlag Berlin Heidelberg; 2014.

2. Branco BC, Naik-Mathuria B, Montero-Baker M, et al. Increasing use of endovascular therapy in pediatric arterial trauma. 2017; 66:1175-1183. doi: 10.1016/j.jvs.2017.04.072.

3. Morão S, Ferreira RS, Camacho N, Vital VP, Pascoal J, Ferreira ME, Capitão LM, Gonçalves FB. Vascular Trauma in Children-Review from a Major Paediatric Center. Ann Vasc Surg. 2018 May; 49:229-233. doi: 10.1016/j.avsg.2017.10.036. Epub 2018 Feb 9. PMID: 29428539.

4. Barmparas G, Inaba K, Talving P, David JS, Lam L, Plurad D, Green D, Demetriades D. Pediatric vs adult vascular trauma: a National Trauma Databank review. J Pediatr Surg. 2010 Jul; 45(7):1404-12. doi: 10.1016/j.jpedsurg.2009.09.017. PMID: 20638516.

5. Rozycki GS, Tremblay LN, Feliciano DV, McClelland WB. Blunt vascular trauma in the extremity: diagnosis, management, and outcome. J Trauma. 2003 Nov; 55(5):814-24. doi: 10.1097/01.TA.0000087807.44105.AE. PMID: 14608150.

6. Whitehouse WM, Coran AG, Stanley JC, Kuhns LR, Weintraub WH, Fry WJ. Pediatric Vascular Trauma: Manifestations, Management, and Sequelae of Extremity Arterial Injury in Patients Undergoing Surgical Treatment. Arch Surg. 1976; 111(11):1269–1275. doi:10.1001/archsurg.1976.01360290103016

7. Klinkner DB, Arca MJ, Lewis BD, Oldham KT, Sato TT. Pediatric vascular injuries: patterns of injury, morbidity, and mortality. J Pediatr Surg. 2007 Jan; 42(1):178-82; discussion 182-3. doi: 10.1016/j.jpedsurg.2006.09.016. PMID: 17208561.

8. Wang SK, Drucker NA, Raymond JL, Rouse TM, Fajardo A, Lemmon GW, Dalsing MC, Gray BW. Long-term outcomes after pediatric peripheral revascularization secondary to trauma

at an urban level I center. J Vasc Surg. 2019 Mar; 69(3):857-862.doi:10.1016/j.jvs.2018.07.029.
Epub 2018 Oct 3. PMID: 30292605.

Clinical case 02

Open forearm trauma with radial pulse abolition complicated by compartment syndrome: a case report.

Introduction :

Open vascular injuries are relatively common and forearm arteries account for 20% of total arterial injuries [1].

They can be life-threatening and functionally disabling for the limbs. They are always associated with lesions of the soft parts or neighbouring organs. The clinical presentation is variable.

The aim of this paper is to report a case of open forearm trauma with radial pulse abolition complicated after surgical repair of compartment syndrome.

Observation:

We report the observation of a 24 year old male with open trauma of the right forearm with associated skin, muscle and vascular breakdown of undetermined mechanism. Physical examination showed active red and black bleeding through an open forearm wound with skin and muscle breakdown associated with abolition of the right radial pulse with coldness of the right hand and forearm associated with a motor deficit of the latter.

Intraoperative exploration revealed transection of all forearm muscles, stretching of the median nerve with total transection of the middle humeral artery associated with approximately 08 cm of arterial loss.

The procedure consisted of restoring arterial continuity through the saphenous vein inverted terminolaterally with partial muscle approximation (Figure 1).

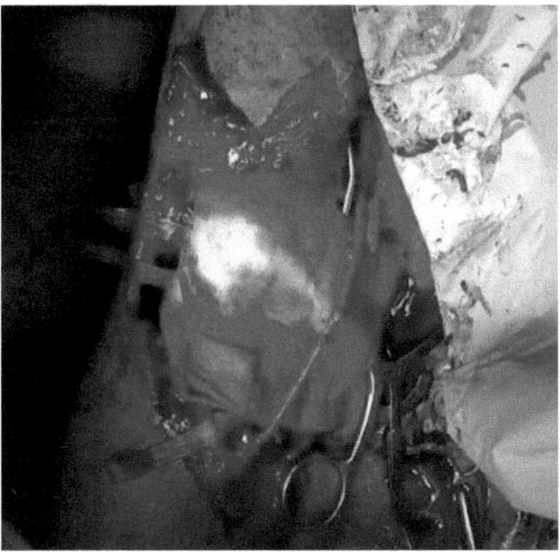

Figure 01: Intraoperative image after revascularisation

Results :

The intraoperative follow-up was marked by a compartment syndrome that benefited from a relief aponevrotomy complicated by parietal sepsis of the right forearm that progressed favourably under antibiotic therapy.

Discussions :

Trauma to the forearm arteries accounts for 20% of all arterial trauma and up to 40% when limited to the upper limb [1-2]. Initially, the trauma may not be perceived because most patients do not show signs of ischaemia [3].

Patients with penetrating forearm trauma should be carefully examined prior to suturing superficial wounds, paying particular attention to signs of vascular injury. Early diagnosis and management not only results in a higher rate of preserved limbs, but also a lower rate of functional impairment of the affected limb [1-3].

As ligation of the radial and ulnar arteries often does not result in significant sequelae, there is little literature on the subject [4].

Reports from the World War II experience, where arterial injuries were treated solely by arterial ligation, show an amputation rate of 5.1% for radial artery injuries, 1.5% for ulnar artery injuries and 39% for concomitant injuries [5]. If only one of the forearm arteries was injured, without signs of ischaemia, it could be ligated with little risk of sequelae [4].

In the presence of ischaemia or concomitant injury to the humeral arteries, arterial restoration must be performed. A reverse saphenous vein graft was performed in our patient [5, 6, 7].

According to McCready, patients with forearm artery injuries rarely require a fasciotomy, which is performed through a large longitudinal incision in the flexor compartment, which can be extended through the carpal ligament into the hand [8].

Walkmann's syndrome can be seen postoperatively requiring a pressure-relief aponevrotomy, as in the case of our patient with compartment syndrome who underwent a pressure-relief aponevrotomy [9].

Conclusion:

Open vascular trauma can result in either haemorrhage or ischaemia. Exploration of the humeral artery should be systematic after open elbow trauma. The presence of a vessel injury should be suspected and explored in the presence of an opening in the path of a vascular axis. The treatment is adapted to the vascular lesions and possibly to the associated lesions. It is conventional surgical or endovascular. The urgency of its implementation depends on the intensity of the haemorrhagic shock or the downstream ischaemic repercussions. Walkman's syndrome may occur postoperatively.

References:

1. Nelson Wolosker Paulo Celso Motta Guimarães Alvaro Gauděncio Sérgio Kuzniec Marcel Scheinman Ricardo Aun Berilo Langer. Sao Paulo Med. J. 112 (1) .Mar 1994. https://doi.org/10.1590/S1516318019940001000002 . Trauma to arteries of the forearm

2. DRAPANAS, T.; HEWITT, R. T.; WEICHERT, R. F. & SMITH, A. D. -Civilian vascular injuries: A critical appraisal of three decades of management. Ann Surg, 172: 351, 1970.

3. TOZZI, F. L.; AUN, R; BECHARA, M. J.; WOLOSKER, N. & WAKSMAN, H. - Arteriografia em pacientes vítimas de trauma em trajeto vascular sem sinal clínico de lesão arterial. Cir Vase Ang, 4: 19, 1988.

4. SITZMAN, J. V. & ERNST, C. B. - Management of arm arterial injuries. Surgery, 96: 896, 1984.

5. DeBAKEY, M. E. & SIMEONE, F. A. - Battle injuries of the arteries in World War II. Ann Surg, 123: 534, 1946.

6. Lakehal R, Bendjaballah S, Aimer F, et al. Total humeral artery transection in open dislocation of the left elbow during a tree fall: about a case. Batna J Med Sci 2017;4(2):169-170. https://doi.org/10.48087/BJMScr.2017.4210

7. Redha Lakehal, Farid Aymer, Soumaya Bendjaballah, et al. 2022. Total section of the humeral artery during a fall on a sharp part of a mirror: Case Report. Clin J Orthop. 4: 01-03.

8. McCREADY, R. A. - Vascular trauma of upper extremity. Surg Clin N Am, 4: 755, 1988.

9. Ricco JB, Fébrer G. Vascular trauma of the limbs. Encycl.Med.Chir. Paris Techniques Chirurgicales Chirurgie Vasculaire, 43- 025 2006.

Clinical case 03

Trauma of the popliteal artery following knee dislocation: a case report.

Introduction :

The combination of knee dislocation and arterial injury is rare, devastating and potentially life-threatening, usually caused by high energy trauma. This association is often seen in polytrauma patients and may progress to ischaemia or even amputation [1,2]. Diagnosis is made by standard radiography of the face and profile. A vascular and neurological assessment is necessary. The vascular lesion is identified by angio-CT of the knee. Immediate treatment is the reduction and treatment of closed vascular lesions [2,3].

We report a case of knee dislocation with occlusion of the popliteal artery in its articular portion complicated by acute ischemia.

Observation:

A 43 year old woman with no profession and no notable pathological history was admitted to the emergency room following intense pain, coldness in the right leg and total functional impotence of the right leg following a dislocation of the right knee secondary to a fall down a flight of stairs. The examination found the patient conscious, cooperative, hemodynamically stable and respiratory. The physical examination noted the absence of deformation and posterior displacement of the right lower limb, the absence of any notion of skin opening, cold right leg and foot with paleness of the toes, the absence of paralysis of the common fibular nerve, abolished popliteal, pedal and tibial pulses. The examination of the contralateral limb was unremarkable. The knee X-ray did not reveal any osteoarticular lesion. The echo-doppler revealed a thrombosis of the popliteal artery.

The patient was operated on under general anaesthesia with tracheal intubation, in the supine position. A medial lateral incision of the right knee was made.

Surgical exploration was not performed until after 15 hours. The popliteal vein and nerve were unharmed but the joint capsule was torn. The popliteal artery was completely severed with retraction of the ends (Figure 01). The procedure consisted of a reverse homolateral saphenous vein bypass implanted between the lower part of the superficial femoral artery and the rest of the popliteal artery (Figure 02) with a proximal and a distal lateral anastomosis.

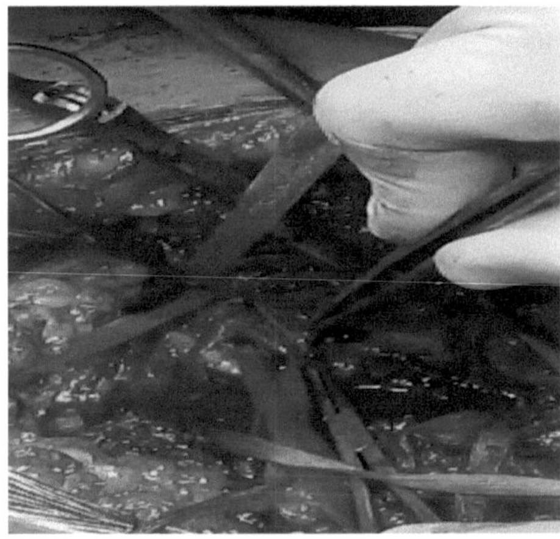

Figure 01: Intraoperative image before arterial repair showing thrombosis of the popliteal artery.

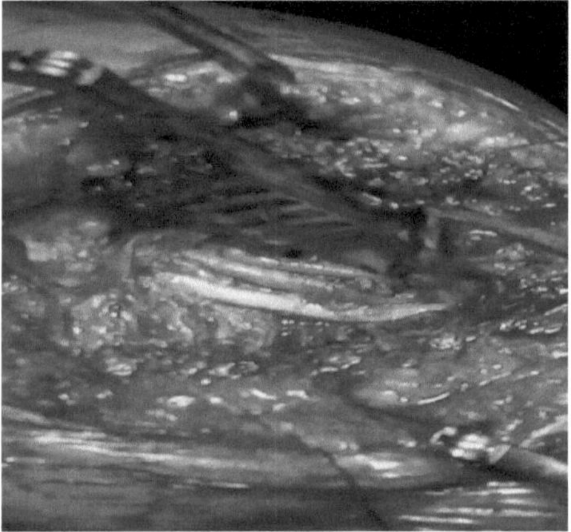

Figure 02: Intraoperative image after arterial repair.

Results :

The length of stay in the intensive care unit was 24 hours and the hospital stay 5 days. The left lower limb is warm and well perfused. No reperfusion-related complications were noted. Postoperative CT angiography showed a patent bypass (Figure 3).

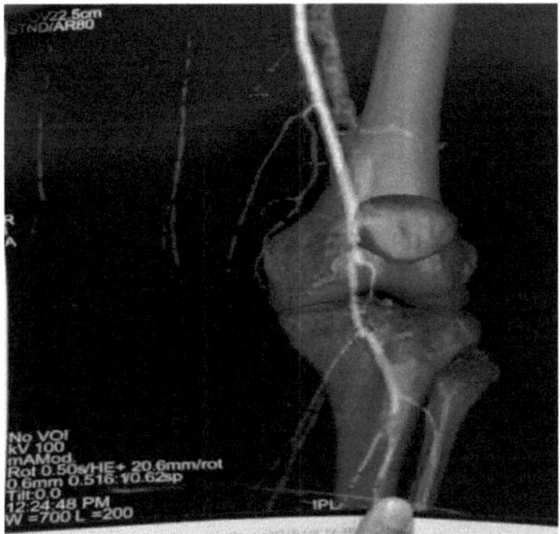

Figure 03: Angioscanographic image of the quality control knee of the arterial repair.

The patient was transferred to the trauma department for treatment of knee instability.

Discussions :

Knee dislocations can be simply defined as "ligamentous injuries with loss of continuity of the tibiofemoral joint" [1]. The association of a popliteal artery injury during a knee dislocation revealed by ischaemia is rare [2]. A popliteal artery injury may initially only affect the intima and therefore will not cause distal ischaemia until the artery subsequently becomes occluded. An undiagnosed arterial injury has a high risk of ischaemic complications, which may lead to amputation [3,7].

Arterial complications are the most serious aspect of knee dislocation. They are frequent and have a highly variable amputation rate, depending on the time taken for revascularisation and the associated lesions. The frequency and severity of arterial lesions mean that they must be investigated in the face of any bi-cross lesion, not only clinically but also systematically by arteriography, as lesions by intimal flap with a perceived pulse may be revealed late (10% to 30% of popliteal involvement with a perceived pulse) [4].

Knee angio-CT of the knee is the reference method for vascular assessment after knee dislocation [3], unfortunately our case did not benefit from this radiological exploration.

The prognosis depends on the speed of management. Vascular repair often involves bypass surgery [5], as in the case of our patient. The initial treatment consisted of emergency joint reduction without fixation, followed by bypass surgery of the popliteal artery via the reversed long saphenous vein. These recognised knee injury associations, treated quickly and conscientiously as a team, lead to a favourable outcome [5,6]. In our patient, the result was favourable with good recovery of the limb.

Conclusion:

Many knee dislocations are accompanied by popliteal artery or nerve damage. Knee dislocations are often under-diagnosed because they are rare and occur as a result of high-energy trauma with embarrassing and potentially fatal injuries. Immediately reduce the dislocated knee and consult a vascular surgeon to repair any vascular damage.

References:

1. R. C. Schenck, D. L. Richter, and D. C. Wascher, "Knee dislocations: lessons learned from 20-year follow-up," Orthopaedic Journal of Sports Medicine, vol. 2, no. 5, pp. 1-10, 2014.

2. Thierno Souleymane Bah et al. Fracture-luxation of the knee with occlusion of the popliteal artery: a case report. PAMJ Clinical Medicine. 2020; 4 (29). 10.11604/pamj-cm.2020.4.29.23775.

3. Vaidya R, Roth M, Nanavati D, Prince M, et al: Low-velocity knee dislocations in obese and morbidly obese patients. Orthop J Sports Med 3 (4):2325967115575719, 2015. doi: 10.1177/2325967115575719.

4. Green NE, Allen BI. Vascular injuries associated with dislocation of the knee. J Bone Joint Surg Am. 1977 Mar; 59 (2): 236-9. PubMed| Google Scholar.

5. P. Bonnevialle et al. Knee injuries associated with popliteal artery rupture: Retrospective study of a series of 54 cases - 18/04/08. Doi: 10.1016/S0035-1040(06)75840-8.

6. Gupta S, Fazal MA, Haddad F. Traumatic anterior knee dislocation and tibial shaft fracture: a case report. Journal of Orthopaedic Surgery. 2007; 15(1): 81-3. PubMed| Google Scholar.

7. N. E. Green and B. L. Allen, "Vascular injuries associated with dislocation of the knee," The Journal of Bone & Joint Surgery-American Volume 59, no. 2, pp. 236-239, 1977.

Clinical case 04

Total transection of the common femoral vein following a cycling accident in a 16-year-old child: a case report.

Introduction :

Vascular injuries to the limbs are fortunately rare in children (about 0.6% of admissions to child trauma). Their rarity is directly related to the lack of research on the subject, but their frequency is increasing with the development of means of locomotion and the rise in the crime rate in an increasingly young population.

The aim of this work is to report a case of total section of the common femoral vein without associated arterial injury following a cycling accident.

Observation:

We report the observation of a 16 year old child who had a bicycle accident resulting in a penetrating wound of the left thigh.

Physical examination showed significant mucocutaneous pallor; enormous swelling of the left Scarpa with two orifices, one on the outer side of the thigh and the other on the homolateral Scarpa, associated with abolished pulses of the corresponding lower limb.

Operative investigation showed a huge Scarpa haematoma compressing the common femoral artery with section of the common femoral vein with loss of venous substance without associated nerve or arterial damage.

The procedure consisted of repairing the vein with the homolateral cephalic vein.

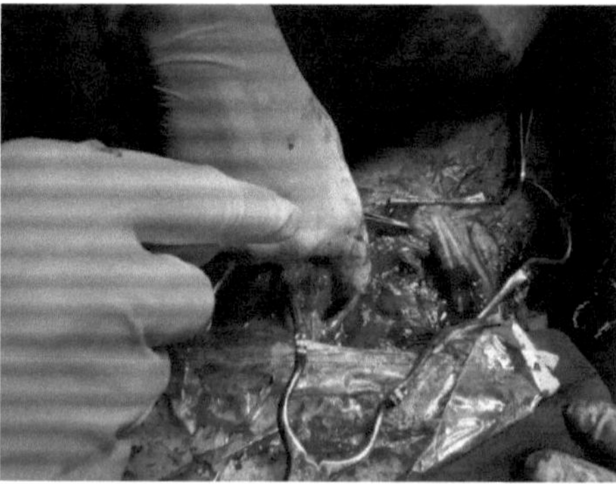

Figure 01: Intraoperative image with restoration of venous continuity.

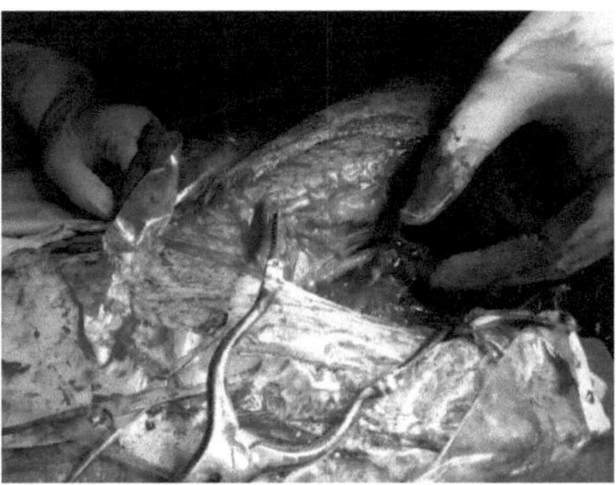

Figure 02: Intraoperative image with restoration of venous continuity.

Results :

Intraoperative follow-up was favourable in terms of revascularisation of the left lower limb with reappearance of the left femoral, popliteal and pedal pulses with warm and mobile limb. Stay in intensive care unit was 01 day. Immediate and medium-term postoperative follow-up was favourable in terms of vitality and function. Venous Doppler ultrasound of the traumatized lower limb showed a permeable montage without anastomotic stenosis or signs of thrombophlebitis.

Discussions :

The most serious complication in this type of accident is thrombophlebitis of the lower limbs, which is why the patient was put on Sintrom for six months.

The loss of femoral venous substance was filled with a vascular substitute: homolateral cephalic vein.

Conclusion:

Vascular trauma in children is a rare reason for surgical consultation. They represent a real threat to the functional prognosis of the limb, especially because of their frequent association with bone, nerve and tendon injuries. This is why it is recommended to systematically perform an imaging test to look for bone, vascular and tissue lesions in a patient outside of any vital emergency context. Knowledge of certain parameters such as the circumstances of the accident can help predict the severity of the injury.

Refernces :

1. Maciej Z, Jakub K, Nicholas I, Marcin G, Zbigniew K. Posttraumatic Reconstruction of External Iliac and Common Femoral Veins Using Femoral Vein Interposition Autograft. Ann Vasc Surg. 2018 Nov; 53:266.e9-266.e11.doi: 10.1016/j.avsg.2018.04.026. Epub 2018 Aug 18. PMID: 30012455.

2. O. Kacimi, A. Idrissi, L. Bahir, A. Siwane, N. Chikhaoui. Vascular trauma of the limbs: Contribution of vascular imaging (about 06 cases). Rev Maroc Chir Orthop Traumato 2007; 32: 35-40.

3. Simms M, Mehat MS, Buckels JA. Phlebology. 2008; 23(5):227-9.doi: 10.1258/phleb.2008.007081. PMID: 18806205.

4. Hu H, Cai Y, Wang C, Yang C, Duan Z, Zhang J, Xin S. Successful treatment of posttraumatic phlegmasia cerulea dolens by reconstructing the external iliac vein: a case report. J Med Case Rep. 2014 May 14;8:149. doi: 10.1186/1752-1947-8-149. PMID: 24885801 .

5. Hobson RW, Yeager RA, Lynch TG, et al. Femoral venous trauma: techniques for surgical management and early results. Am J Surg 1983;146:220-4.

6. Manley NR, Magnotti LJ, Fabian TC, Croce MA, Sharpe JP. Impact of venorrhaphy and vein ligation in isolated lower-extremity venous injuries on venous thromboembolism and edema. J Trauma Acute Care Surg. 2018 Feb;84(2):325-329.doi: 10.1097/TA.0000000000001746. PMID: 29370050 .

7. Z. L. Randimbinirina, T. Rajaobelison, F. F. Randrianarisoa, M.L.A.Ravalisoa, A.J.C Rakotoarisoa. Post-traumatic peripheral vascular wounds in the Joseph Ravoahangy Andrianavalona. Rev. Anesthesia-Reanim. Med. Urg. Toxicol. 2018 (January-June); 10(1): 1-4.

Clinical case 05

Aortic wound during reoperation: a case report.

Introduction :

Thoracic aortic wounds are exceptional lesions with a particularly high mortality if immediate medical and surgical management is not provided [1]. Aortic wounds during cardiac redux surgery are exceptional. Diagnosis is based on intraoperative exploration. The prognosis is poor [7]. Treatment is based on surgery.

The aim of this observation is to raise awareness among residents and young cardiac surgeons of the seriousness of this incident during cardiac surgery.

Observation:

We report the observation of a young man aged 35 years, operated 21 years ago for sub-valvular aortic stenosis presenting for a few months with exertional dyspnoea and syncopes, hospitalised for surgical management of a recurrent and symptomatic sub-valvular aortic stenosis.

Chest X-ray profile showed a small space between the heart and the sternum.

The ECG showed a regular sinus rhythm with left ventricular hypertrophy.

Echocardiography showed subvalvular aortic narrowing on circumferential membrane: LV: 54/32 mm, PAPS: 70 mm hg, EF: 70%.

After iterative sternotomy, an aortic wound occurred during the removal of steel wire expressed by a clear jet of red blood, after heparinisation, closure of the sternum on an inflated Foley catheter introduced into the aortic wound and installation of a femoral-femoral extracorporeal circulation (ECP) to compensate for blood loss in normothermia.

Intraoperative exploration after retro sternal dissection a frank wound of the ascending aorta of about 01/01 cm controlled by partial aortic clamping (Figures 1,2).

The procedure consisted of a two-strip Teflon overlay repair of the aortic wound.

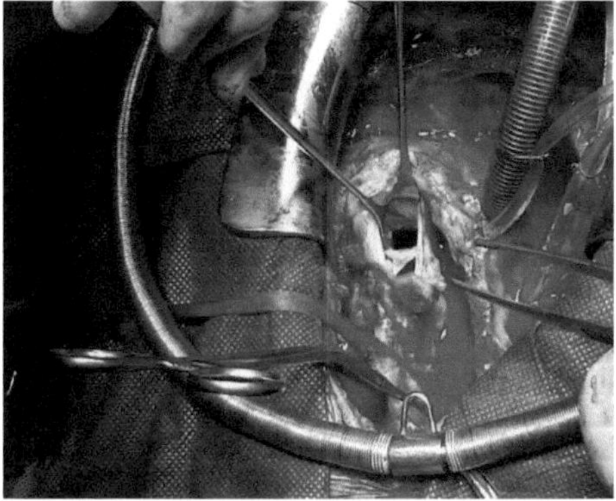

Figure 01: Intraoperative image of the aortic wound

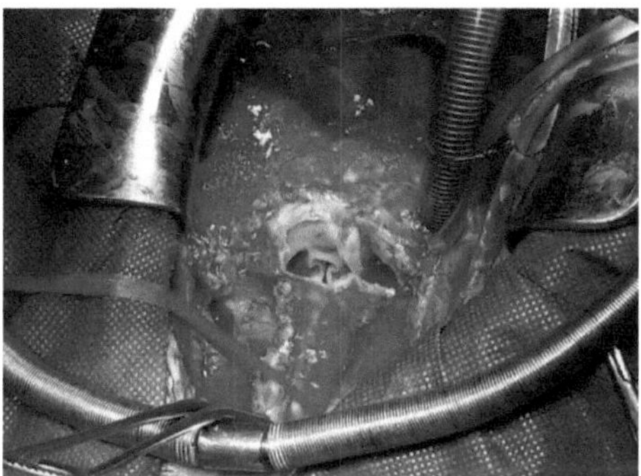

Figure 02: Intraoperative image of the aortic wound

Discussion:

Anatomically, the ascending thoracic aorta, strictly retrosternal, is the portion between the aortic orifice and the brachiocephalic artery trunk. It is approximately 3-5 cm long and is contained within the pericardial sac with the pulmonary artery [2].

Epidemiologically, thoracic aortic wounds are reported as isolated cases in the literature. Their prevalence is therefore very low: only 1% of bullet wounds [3]. The largest series collected 27 patients over a period of 8 years in a single North American centre [4].

Penetrating trauma is the cause in 82% of cases [5]. Firearms were the invading agent in 69% of cases and knives in 18% of cases [6]. Exceptionally, iatrogenic injuries to the ascending aorta during angiography [5] and by the tip of a vertebral screw for spinal osteosynthesis or to the aortic arch during placement of a central subclavian line [5] have been described. No observation of a wound of the aorta during a sternotomy has been published as in the case of our patient.

Reoperations in cardiac surgery are not without complications, especially bleeding complications: right ventricular, right atrial and aortic wounds.

Clinically, a distinction is made between haemodynamically stable "aortic injuries" and unstable injuries (systolic blood pressure < 90 mm Hg), which are the most common, with collapse occurring in 82.5% of cases [1,6]. Haemodynamically unstable patients should be treated surgically immediately in order to achieve haemostasis as soon as possible [6].

We insist on the interest of leaving the two scarpas triangles free in case of redux and on the presence of a blood recovery system (Cell Saver®), in order to quickly compensate for blood loss in case of intraoperative bleeding accidents. It is also necessary to respect all the rules of re-intervention in cardiac surgery such as the CEC circuit unblocked on the operating field and heparin prepared on the operating table.

The mortality of aortic wounds remains particularly high, above 90%, despite the progress made in the emergency management of these injuries [7]. Thus, for many authors, only the prevention of these injuries could improve survival.

The originality of our observation lies in the mechanism of the aortic wound, never described before, and in its favourable evolution, made possible by immediate medical and surgical management, the absence of associated lesions, and the absence of prolonged collapse. This observation perfectly illustrates the risk of serious complications of sterotomy during reoperations, which can be the cause of cardiac or large vessel wounds, the mortality of which remains above 50%.

Conclusion:

This observation shows a serious and exceptional but often lethal intraoperative incident. It requires rapid and effective surgical management. The prevention of penetrating lesions of the thoracic aorta during cardiac surgery is a way to reduce their mortality. It requires training and supervision of residents and young cardiac surgeons. A good knowledge of anatomical relationships and the respect of general safety rules should reduce the risk of complications.

Reference :

1. J. Jarry, L. Lang-Lazdunski, j.-P. Perez, R. Barthelemy, O. Berets, R. Jancovici Presse Med 2004, 33:22-4 © 2004, Masson, Paris

2. Rouvière H, Delmas A. Aorta. In: Anatomie humaine : Tronc. Editions Masson, Paris, 1997; 169.

3. Cornwell EE, Kennedy F. Gunshot wounds to the thoracic aorta in the 90s: Only prevention will make a difference. Am Surg 1995; 61:721-3.

4. Pate JW, Cole FH. Penetrating injuries of the aortic arch and its branches. Ann Thorac Surg 1993;55:586-92.

5. Weaver FA, Suda RW. Injuries to the ascending aorta, aortic arch and great vessels. Surg Gynec Obstet 1989;169:27-31.

6. Demetriades D. Penetrating injuries to the thoracic great vessels. J Cardiac Surg 1997;12:173-80.

7. Endara SA, Xabregas AA. Major mediastinal injury from crossbow bolt. *Ann Thorac Surg* 2001;72:2107-9.

Clinical case 06

Total transection of the lower humeral artery and median nerve in a girl during a suicide attempt: a case report.

Introduction :

Ballistic trauma is as much a wartime pathology as a peacetime one [1]. The pathophysiology of ballistic trauma is based on the behaviour of the projectile in the body. High velocity firearm injuries are unique to the military. Low-velocity firearm injuries are more commonly encountered in civilian settings. Whilst haemorrhage is the primary cause of early death, infection is the second most common cause by the twenty-fourth hour. The management of a patient suffering from ballistic trauma is an infrequent reason for recourse to emergency medicine and more particularly to out-of-hospital care [1]. Secondary complications, particularly septic complications, and the seriousness of associated injuries such as haemorrhagic processes, require an assessment and prioritisation involving mobile emergency and resuscitation teams.

The aim of this work is to report a case of total transection of the lower humeral artery and median nerve with loss of substance in a girl during a suicide attempt.

Observation:

We report the observation of a 16 year old girl with psychiatric disorders since childhood under antidepressant treatment who suffered a ballistic trauma of the left upper limb during a suicide attempt. Physical examination of the left upper limb showed the absence of active bleeding with abolition of the radial pulse, coldness and pallor of the left hand and forearm associated with a sensitivomotor deficit of the latter two, the rest of the physical examination was without particularity with blood pressure at 80/50 mm HG.

Chest X-ray showed a TIA of 0.50.

Bone radiography of the left upper limb was unremarkable.

ECG was in regular sinus rhythm

After an emergency assessment, the patient was operated on under general anaesthesia and endotracheal intubation.

Intraoperative exploration revealed, in addition to the entry and exit ports in the arm, a total section of the lower humeral artery with loss of arterial substance as well as total section of the median nerve and retraction of the proximal end without muscular section of the left arm and without finding a projectile during trimming.

After trimming and washing, the procedure consisted of restoring humeral arterial continuity by means of a reverse saphenous vein implanted lateroterminally between the two arterial ends (Figures 01, 02), with the two nerve ends marked out so as to facilitate their identification during a future operation.

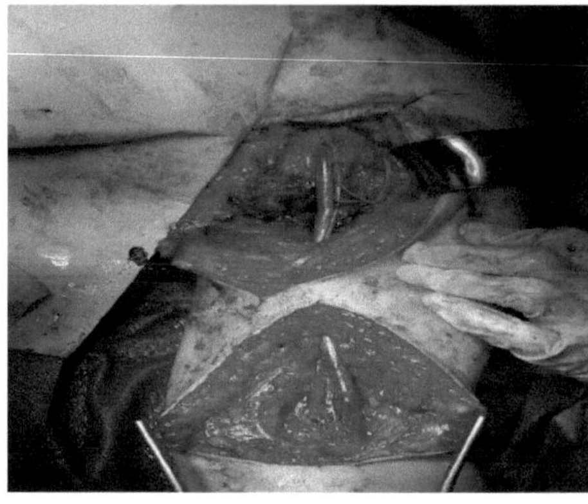

Figure 01: Intraoperative image with restoration of arterial continuity.

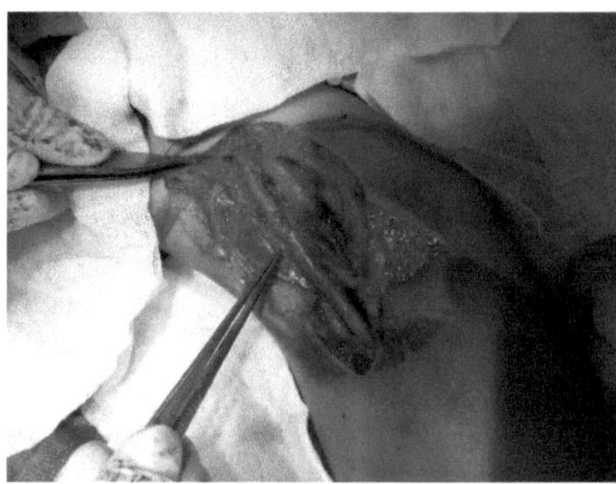

Figure 02: Intraoperative image with restoration of arterial continuity.

Results :

The length of stay in the intensive care unit was 24 hours. The postoperative course was favourable in terms of revascularisation of the upper limb with persistence of paralysis of the left hand and forearm. A follow-up CT angiogram of the traumatized limb showed a patent montage without anastomotic stenosis (Figure 03). The patient was referred to her attending psychiatrist for psychiatric management and to specialist neurological surgery centres.

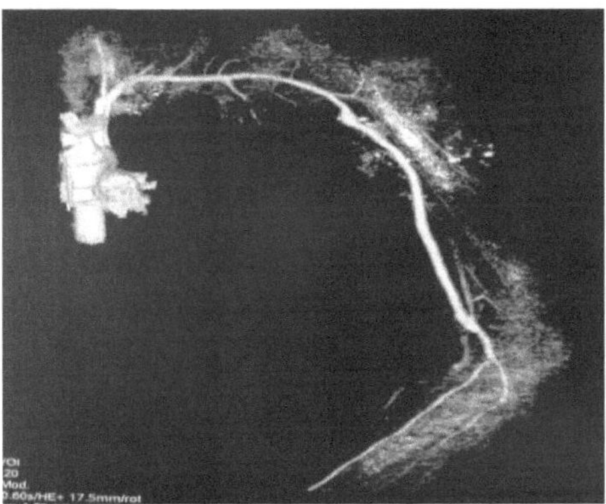

Figure 03: Postoperative angioscannographic monitoring

Discussions :

According to Laforge [2], in civil practice, 48% of ballistic injuries are due to aggression, 47% to suicide and 3% to accidents. In our patient, the circumstances of the accident were suicide. Among 39 patients treated by Dakouré [3] for ballistic trauma, 58.9% had been accidentally injured.

Ballistic trauma is a real public health problem in many countries, especially in the developing world [3]. In 2011, in Burkina Faso, a study conducted by Mzida and colleagues on firearm injuries found that the upper limbs were affected in 18.5% and the lower limbs in 51.8% [5].

The absence of foreign bodies in the wound indicated that it was a bullet and not a shrapnel, and the limitation of soft tissue damage showed that the bullet had a high energy at its exit point that spread the soft tissue [6-8].

The loss of humeral arterial substance was filled by a vascular substitute: a reversed saphenous vein taken from the homolateral thigh after verification of the arterial axes by fogarty probe and implanted latero-terminally. The absence of surgery on the median nerve was due to the extent of the neurological damage with a 10 cm loss of substance and retraction of the proximal end of the median nerve.

Intraoperative follow-up was favourable in terms of revascularisation of the left upper limb with persistence of paralysis of the hand and left forearm. The immediate and medium-term postoperative follow-up was favourable in terms of vitality and vascularisation but unfavourable in terms of neurology. The CT angiography of the traumatized limb showed a permeable montage without anastomotic stenosis [9].

The severity of the associated injuries requires assessment and prioritisation by mobile emergency and resuscitation teams at the site of the ballistic trauma, which was not the case for our patient. The evacuation was carried out without assessment or prioritisation from a hospital in the periphery to a cardiovascular surgery centre, passing through three non-specialised hospital structures during the journey. The journey time was more than 15 hours.

The patient requires psychiatric care to prevent further suicide attempts.

Conclusion:

Ballistic trauma in children is a rare reason for surgical consultation. However, certain pitfalls should not be overlooked and significant internal injuries should be contrasted with a non-traumatic entry point. This is why it is recommended to systematically carry out an imaging test to look for bone, vascular and tissue lesions in a patient outside the context of any vital emergency. Knowledge of certain parameters such as the circumstances of the accident and the type of firearm used can help predict the severity of the injuries. Ballistic trauma is a surgical emergency that must be treated as soon as possible to avoid complications.

References :

1. Lamah L, Keita D, Marie Camara I, Lamine Bah M, Sory S, Diallo MM. Ballistic Trauma of Limbs. Open Orthop J. 2017;11:268-273. Published 2017 Mar 31. doi:10.2174/1874325001711010268

2. Laforge V., Del Nista D. Ballistic injuries in civil practice. Reanoxyo. 2008;23:25-26. [Google Scholar].

3. Dakoure P.W.H., Abalo A.G., Sanon B.G., Da S.C., Some O.R., Kambou T., Ouedraog R.K. Ballistic Injuries in Bobo-Dioulasso University Hospital (Burkina Faso): About 39 cases. J. Sci. Res. Lomé 2011; 13(4):1-4. [Google Scholar].

4. Ly L. War injuries the epidemio-clinical and therapeutic aspects of war wounded in the department of Orthopaedic and Traumatological Surgery at the University Hospital of Pr Bocar Sidi Sall of Kati. FMOS medical thesis; Bamako; 2018.

5. Zida M, Diallo O, Zan A, Traoré SS. Gunshot wounds from the 2011 military insurgency in Ouagadougou (BURKINA FASO).

6. Volgas D.A., Stannard J.P., Alonso J.E. Current orthopaedic treatment of ballistic injuries. Injury. 2005;36(3):380-386. doi: 10.1016/j.injury.2004.08.038. [PubMed] [CrossRefGoogle Scholar] []

7. Fackler M.L., Malinowski J.A. The wound profile: a visual method for quantifying gunshot wound components. J. Trauma. 1985;25(6):522-529. doi: 10.1097/00005373-198506000-00009. [PubMed] [CrossRef] [Google Scholar]

8. Giannou C., Baldan M. War surgery. Vol. 1. Geneva Switzerland: International Committee of the Red Cross; 2010. pp. 57-95. [Google Scholar]

9. A. Daghfous , K. Bouzaïdi , M. Abdelkefi , S. Rebai , A. Zoghlemi , M. Mbarek , L. Rezgui Marhoul. Contribution of imaging in the initial management of ballistic trauma ; Journal of Diagnostic and Interventional Radiology ; Volume 96, 2015.

Clinical case 07

Total section of the humeral artery by an iron bar during a fall from a scaffold: a case report.

Introduction :

Vascular injuries are injuries that involve a vessel, either an artery or a vein or both. They can be open or closed. Open limb vascular injuries are relatively common. Vascular trauma of the limbs is the most predominant (90%).the aetiological circumstances have changed in recent years in peacetime (public road accidents, iatrogenic trauma, etc.).they can affect the functional and vital prognosis of the limbs. They are always associated with lesions of the soft parts or neighbouring organs. The clinical presentation is variable. The aim of this work is to show the interest of surgically exploring the humeral artery as well as the humeral bifurcation during penetrating trauma of the elbow with abolition of the radial pulse.

Observation:

We report the observation of a young 21 year old bricklayer who suffered a penetrating trauma of the left elbow by an iron bar following a fall from a scaffold. He presented an abolition of the left radial pulse without any bone lesion during the physical examination with a well coloured hand and left forearm without any sensitivomotor disorders.

The patient underwent emergency surgery without Doppler ultrasound or arteriography of the upper limb.

Intraoperative exploration showed, after removal of the iron bar, a loss of humeral arterial substance of 03 cm in length with retracted and thrombosed ends without associated nerve or vein damage.

The procedure consisted of restoring humeral arterial continuity via the homolateral basilic vein after preparation of the humeral arterial extremities and verification of a very good flow in the humeral artery and good reflux of the left radial and ulnar arteries.

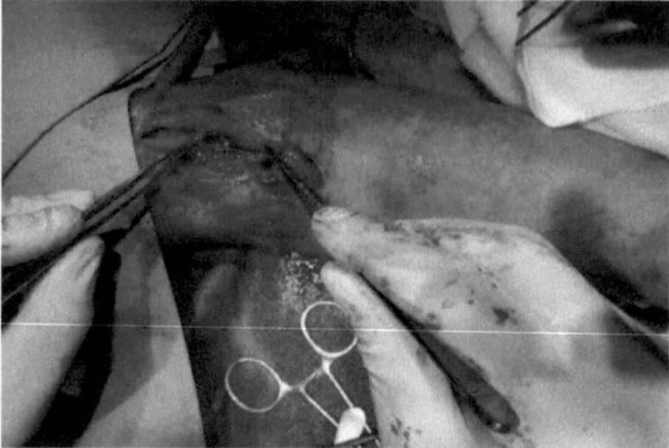

Figure 01: Total transection of the humeral artery by an iron bar with humeral arterial loss of substance but without associated bone, vein or nerve damage.

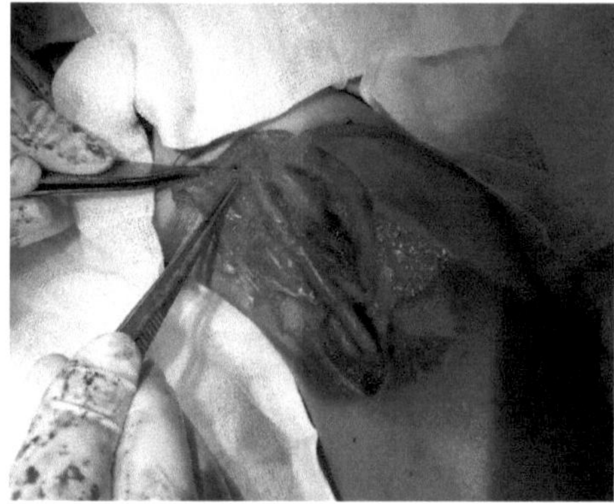

Figure 02: Repair of arterial loss through the homolateral cephalic vein.

Results :

The immediate postoperative course was simple with

-Reappearance of the left radial pulse.

-Sensitivity and motor skills of the limb are retained.

-Warm and colourful member.

The patient is discharged on 03ème postoperative day.

Control echodopplers of the left upper limb performed at 1^{ier} and 3ème months were unremarkable.

Discussion:

Vascular trauma in civil practice always represents a surgical emergency that puts at risk the immediate vital prognosis of the patients but also the functional prognosis of the limbs concerned due to the associated lesions but also due to the lesions induced by the ischaemia. Their management must begin at the scene of the accident by controlling the haemorrhage and early volemic compensation. The assessment of vascular lesions should not focus on obvious lesions such as external haemorrhage but also take into account the possibility of tiered lesions. The quality of the initial assessment will lead to appropriate management which may include open and endoluminal surgery depending on the type and location of the vascular lesions. A vascular wound of the humeral artery may go unnoticed, hence the interest of a careful examination of the traumatized limb in the case of any penetrating trauma of the latter, as in the case of our patient.

The management of associated lesions will be discussed with all the actors concerned with a view to multidisciplinary management.
The type of repair of the vascular injury depends on the nature of the injury. [9]

The basilic vein can be used instead of the saphenous vein to compensate for arterial loss. [7-8-9]

Conclusion:

Open vascular trauma can result in either haemorrhage or ischaemia. [1-2-3]

Exploration of the humeral artery should be systematic after penetrating elbow trauma with pulse suppression. [9]

The presence of a vessel lesion must be suspected and explored in the presence of an opening in the path of a vascular axis. [9]

The treatment is adapted to the vascular lesions and possibly to associated lesions. It is conventional or endovascular surgery. [1]

The urgency of its implementation depends on the intensity of the haemorrhagic shock or the downstream ischemic repercussions. [4-5]

Walkmann's syndrome can occur postoperatively. [1]

References :

1. J.B. Ricco, G. Fébrer. -Vascular trauma of the limbs. Encycl.Med.Chir. Paris
Surgical Techniques Vascular Surgery, 43-025 2006. Article describing the different
anatomopathological aspects of vascular lesions, their mechanisms and their surgical
management.

2. Under the direction of Kieffer E. Traumatismes artériels. Editions AERCV.1995
Focus on vascular trauma.

3. N.M. Rich, P. Rhee. -An historical tour of vascular injury management: from its inception
to the new millennium. Surg Clin North Am 2001; 81: 1199-215. Historical overview of the
management of vascular trauma, and the various works that led to the development of vascular
trauma surgery.

4. O.Doody, M.F.Given, S.M.Lyon . -Extremities- indications and techniques for treatment of
extremity vascular Injuries . Injury 2008; 39: 1295-1303. Review article discussing the recent
use of CT angiography in the diagnosis of vascular injuries and the role of other non-invasive
examinations.

5. Drapanas T, Hewitt RL, Weichert RF, Smith AD. Civilian vascular injuries: a critical
appraisal of three decades of management. Ann Surg 1970; 171: 351 -360.

6.Rich NM: Vascular trauma in Vietnam. J Cardiovasc Surg 1970; 11: 368-377.

7. Rich NM, Baugh JM, Hughes CW. Acute arterial injuries in Vietnam: 1 000 cases.
J Trauma; 1970; 10: 359-369.

8. Orcutt MB, Levin BA, Gastrill HV. Civilian vascular trauma of the upper extremity.
J Trauma 1986; 26: 63-67.

9. Pailler JL, Baranger B, Chemla E, General principles of surgical treatment of arterial trauma of the limbs in E. Kieffer Traumatismes Artériels , Editions AERCV Paris 1995 :45-54.

Clinical case 08

Total humeral artery transection in open dislocation of the left elbow in a tree fall: a case report.

Introduction :

Open vascular trauma is relatively common. They can affect the functional and vital prognosis of the limbs. They are always associated with injuries to the soft tissues or neighbouring organs, and the clinical presentation is variable. The aim of this work is to show an open dislocation of the left elbow associated with a total section of the humeral artery following a fall from a tree.

Observation*:*

We report the observation of a 15 year old girl who fell from a tree with an open dislocation of the left elbow associated with a fracture of the lower extremity of the forearm with abolition of the left radial pulse with well coloured hand and left forearm without sensitivomotor disorders.

The patient underwent emergency surgery without Doppler ultrasound or arteriography of the left upper limb.

Intraoperative exploration showed a 03 cm long loss of left humeral arterial substance with retracted and thrombosed arterial stubs associated with median nerve stretch and complete dislocation of the elbow with rupture of the joint capsule without associated venous injury.

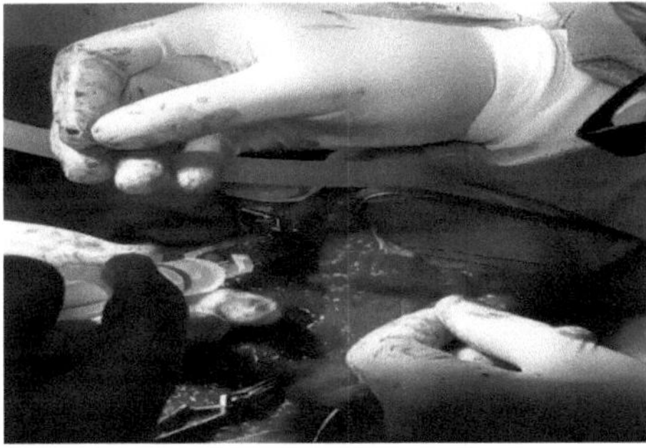

Figure 01: Total transection of the humeral artery in open elbow dislocation.

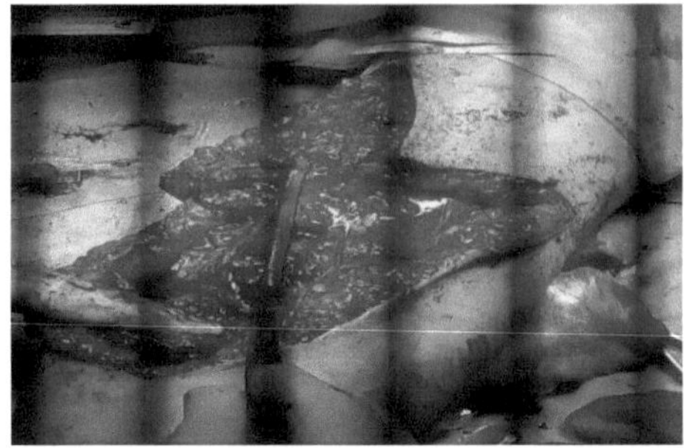

Figure 02 : Repair of arterial loss of substance with a terminally interposed reverse saphenous graft.

The procedure consisted of suturing the joint capsule, re-establishing humeral arterial continuity via the reverse saphenous vein after preparation of the humeral arterial extremities and finally reducing the dislocation of the elbow and the lower extremity of the forearm and immobilising the upper limb with a plaster cast.

Results :

The postoperative course was simple after 24 hours with the appearance of a forearm compartment syndrome requiring a forearm aponeurotomy with a clear improvement afterwards.

-Reappearance of the left radial pulse.

-Sensitivity and motor skills of the left upper limb retained.

-Left upper limb warm and well coloured.

The patient is discharged on 08ème day.

The echodoppler checks of the left upper limb performed on 1^{ier} and 3ème months were unremarkable.

Discussion:

Vascular trauma in civil practice always represents a surgical emergency that puts at risk the immediate vital prognosis of the patients but also the functional prognosis of the limbs concerned due to the associated lesions but also due to the lesions induced by the ischaemia.

Their management must begin at the scene of the accident by controlling the haemorrhage and early volemic compensation. The assessment of vascular lesions should not focus on obvious lesions such as external haemorrhage but also take into account the possibility of tiered lesions. The quality of the initial assessment will result in an adapted management which may include, depending on the type and location of the vascular lesions, open surgery and endoluminal surgery.

The management of associated lesions will be discussed with all the actors concerned with a view to multidisciplinary management.

The association of a vascular lesion with an open bone dislocation is frequent.

The type of repair of the vascular injury depends on the nature of the injury. [7]

Conclusion:

Open vascular trauma can result in either haemorrhage or ischaemia [4-5]. Exploration of the humeral artery should be systematic after open elbow dislocation.

The presence of a vessel lesion should be suspected and explored in the presence of an opening in the path of a vascular axis. [2-3]

Treatment is tailored to the vascular lesions and possibly associated lesions. [9]

It is either conventional or endovascular surgery. The urgency of its implementation depends on the intensity of the haemorrhagic shock or the downstream ischemic repercussions. [1-8-9]

Walkmann's syndrome may occur postoperatively requiring discharge fasciotomies. [8]

References :

1. J.B. Ricco, G. Fébrer. -Vascular trauma of the limbs. Encycl.Med.Chir. Paris
Surgical Techniques Vascular Surgery, 43-025 2006. Article describing the different anatomopathological aspects of vascular lesions, their mechanisms and their surgical management.

2. Under the direction of Kieffer E. Traumatismes artériels. Editions AERCV.1995
Focus on vascular trauma.

3. N.M. Rich, P. Rhee. -An historical tour of vascular injury management: from its inception to the new millennium. Surg Clin North Am 2001; 81: 1199-215. Historical overview of the management of vascular trauma, and the various works that led to the development of vascular trauma surgery.

4. O.Doody, M.F.Given, S.M.Lyon. -Extremities- indications and techniques for treatment of extremity vascular Injuries. Injury 2008; 39: 1295-1303. Review article discussing the recent use of CT angiography in the diagnosis of vascular injuries and the role of other non-invasive examinations.

5. Drapanas T, Hewitt RL, Weichert RF, Smith AD. Civilian vascular injuries: a critical appraisal of three decades of management. Ann Surg 1970; 171: 351 -360.

6. Rich NM: Vascular trauma in Vietnam. J Cardiovasc Surg 1970; 11: 368-377.

7. Rich NM, Baugh JM, Hughes CW. Acute arterial injuries in Vietnam: 1 000 cases.
J Trauma; 1970; 10: 359-369.

8. Orcutt MB, Levin BA, Gastrill HV. Civilian vascular trauma of the upper extremity.
J Trauma 1986; 26: 63-67.

9. Pailler JL, Baranger B, Chemla E, Princpes généraux du traitement chirurgical des traumatismes artériels des membres in E. Kieffer Traumatismes Artériels, Editions AERCV Paris 1995 :45-54.

CONTENTS

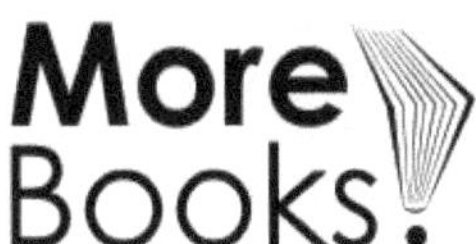

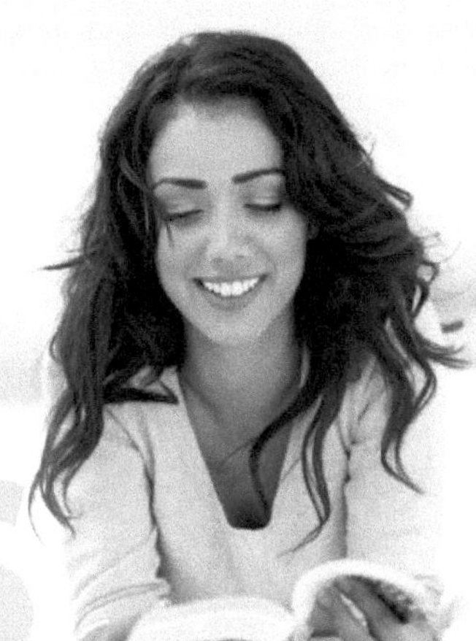

I want morebooks!

Buy your books fast and straightforward online - at one of world's fastest growing online book stores! Environmentally sound due to Print-on-Demand technologies.

Buy your books online at
www.morebooks.shop

Kaufen Sie Ihre Bücher schnell und unkompliziert online – auf einer der am schnellsten wachsenden Buchhandelsplattformen weltweit! Dank Print-On-Demand umwelt- und ressourcenschonend produziert.

Bücher schneller online kaufen
www.morebooks.shop

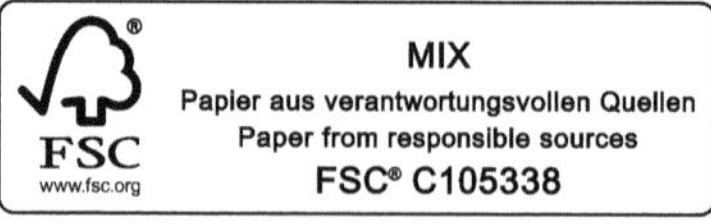

Printed by Books on Demand GmbH, Norderstedt / Germany